Mediterranean diet cookbook on a budget

The ultimate recipe cookbook, which can prevent diseases, lose weight quickly and get lean with amazing and delicious Mediterranean recipes

Richard Colley

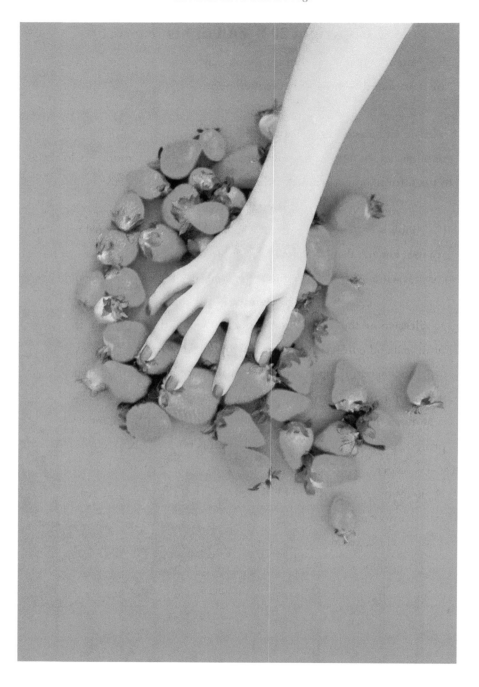

Table of Contents

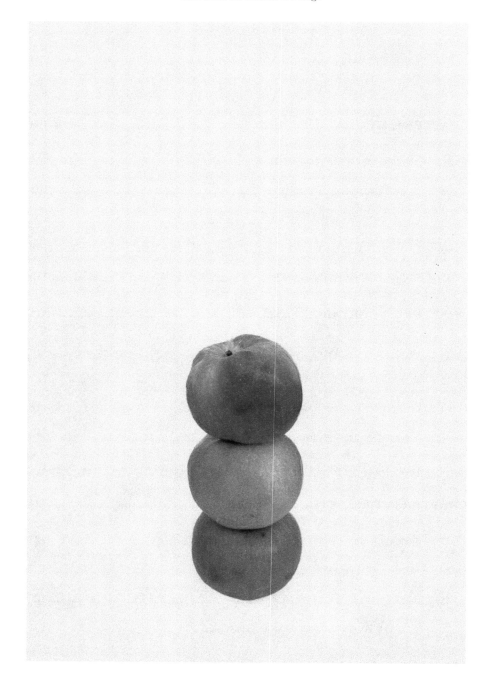

Introduction

The Mediterranean diet claims that lots of fat and relaxation will keep you healthy. If you choose to drop the pounds and keep them off, you will discover the Mediterranean style is the cure you have been seeking. This diet is a fresh way of life. You're ultimately going to want to become familiar with the Mediterranean diet.

The Mediterranean diet is an easy diet to follow. It is an easy diet. The Mediterranean diet is really simple in its approach. Wealthy Italians live longer than many other people on the earth. The Mediterranean diet provides a range of health benefits. Naturally, the Mediterranean diet has lots of influence from France and Italy.

Several medical studies were performed on the Mediterranean diet and found a low incidence of heart disease among men who lived in Crete, one of the regions where this diet was initially used. This diet's main ingredients are fresh fruit, vegetables, olive oil, beans, and herbs. Several other studies found that this Mediterranean diet can significantly reduce stroke incidence and mortality from hypertension.

Studies were also conducted to examine the effects of this diet on the skin of those who followed this diet. It was found that this diet helped to block the development of skin wrinkling and also reduced the incidence of skin cancer in people who followed it. This diet is also excellent for the arteries and lowers the so-called clogged arteries that everyone is afraid of.

The Mediterranean diet is one of my favorites because it is so delicious. Your success when following this diet comes down to the true straightforward nature of this diet. In all reality, there is no fasting, you have to consume every day. They will attempt to relieve their health issues in different ways. It is possible to enjoy a very healthy diet with this. This fat-banishing Mediterranean diet can be used by anybody.

The Mediterranean diet is beneficial for your physical health. It's a fantastic way to live. It's an excellent choice for promoting weight reduction, the treatment of disease, and overall health.

An added benefit is that you can get pleasure from foods you adore while losing weight. Clearly, the extra benefits you get from exercise, the greater you'll stick with it. In the end, the more advantages you get from exercise, the greater you'll stick with it. If you prefer to be as healthy as you can, you have to start by adopting a Mediterranean diet. Exposure to sunlight is good for your health. A healthy lifestyle is great for your existence. A healthy lifestyle is great for the lifespan. The Mediterranean diet is good for your existence. It is a good idea to use the physical strategy on how you want to come to be cured.

The Mediterranean way is the ideal way to cure any kind of health problem When the term Mediterranean diet was first publicly discussed in the United States in the 1970s, it actually referred to a way of preparing food that was healthy and also delicious. Today, however, the term refers to a scientific diet that was originally used many thousands of years ago in the Mediterranean region.

It is important to realize that the Mediterranean diet originally had nothing to do with the reduction of heart disease. It was created before the development of heart disease in humans. This diet was created by humans who had no knowledge of heart disease and obviously didn't think that they were dealing with a disease. There were no such concepts as diet or food at that time. It was a beautiful and very unique way of life. It was set up on the farms which were very large and had fields, orchards, vineyards, walnut groves and olive groves on them. The people ate fresh fruit, nuts, fresh vegetables, herbs and spices. They raised their own meat and milk products. They raised their own grains and rarely even ate much wheat. They ate a variety of meats, especially lamb, goat, turkey, pork. Basic spices were used to flavor food as well. There was no need to make a variety of complex sauces since there was fresh and abundant produce available. The more foods were cooked and processed, the more people developed illnesses that are associated with excessive cooked and processed foods.

It was found that the primitive Mediterranean diet was one of the best, if not the best diet that was available, and it was much better than modern diets.

CHAPTER 1:

Basic Principles of The Diet

Learn How to Understand Nutrition Labels

Look for Short Ingredient List: The bulk of the food is listed according to weight and is usually the first ingredient. If you don't recognize an ingredient, place it back on the shelf! Consider using products that have no more than five ingredients. The longer ingredients probably are the result of unnecessary extras, including artificial preservatives.

Check Serving Sizes: Packages often time contain more than a single serving. Visualize how many calories and the amount of sugar is in a single container. Thus, you need to check the serving size first.

Discover Calorie Counts: It is essential to check the label's calorie count since it is essential during your process using the Mediterranean diet plan.

Avoid Fats: It's important to remove foods from your diet plan that contain any fully hydrogenated or partially hydrogenated oils.

Check the Percent of Daily Value: The daily value will tell you how many nutrients are in each serving of a packaged item.

Get More of These Nutrients: Look for calcium, iron, fiber, vitamin A, and vitamin C.

The Label Explained

- Serving Information at the Top: This provides the size of one serving and per container.
- Check the total calories per serving and container.
- Limit certain nutrients from your diet.
- Provide yourself with plenty of beneficial nutrients
- Understand the % of daily value section.

Avoid These Foods

- Added Sugar: Ice cream, candy, regular soda, plus many others.
- Refined Oils: Canola oil, cottonseed oil, soybean oil, etc.

- Trans fats: Found in various processed foods such as margarine, added sugar, ice cream, candies, table sugar, soda, etc. Added sugars, sugar-sweetened beverages, refined grains, processed meats, and other highly processed foods.
- Processed Meat Products: Hot dogs, processed sausages, bacon
- Refined Grains: Pasta made with refined wheat, white bread

Note If You Are Pregnant: You should avoid some of the oily fish such as swordfish, shark, and tuna because some may contain low levels of toxic heavy metals.

What to Eat Rarely:

- Red meats (Limit to once each week)

Foods You Can Eat

Seafood and Fish: Mussels, clams, crab, prawns, oysters, shrimp, tuna, mackerel, salmon, trout, sardines, anchovies, and more

Poultry: Turkey, duck, chicken, and more

Eggs: Duck, quail, and chicken eggs

Dairy Products: Contain calcium, B12, and Vitamin A: Greek yogurt, regular yogurt, cheese, plus others

Tubers: Yams, turnips, potatoes, sweet potatoes, etc.

Vegetables: Another excellent choice for fiber and antioxidants: Cucumbers, carrots, Brussels sprouts, tomatoes, onions, broccoli, cauliflower, spinach, kale, eggplant, artichokes, fennel, etc.

Seeds and Nuts: Provide minerals, vitamins, fiber, and protein: Macadamia nuts, cashews, pumpkin seeds, sunflower seeds, hazelnuts, chestnuts, Brazil nuts, walnuts, almonds, pumpkin seeds, sesame, poppy, and more

Fruits: Excellent vitamin C choices, antioxidants, and fiber: Peaches, bananas, apples, figs, dates, pears, oranges, strawberries, melons, grapes, etc.

Spices and Herbs: Cinnamon, garlic, pepper, nutmeg, rosemary, sage, mint, basil, parsley, etc.

Whole Grains: Whole grain bread and pasta, buckwheat, whole wheat, barley, corn, whole oats, rye, quinoa, bulgur, couscous

Legumes: Provide vitamins, fiber, carbohydrates, and protein: Chickpeas, pulses, beans, lentils, peanuts, peas

Healthy Fats: Avocado oil, avocados, and olives are excellent fats. The monounsaturated fat which is found in olive oil is a fat that can help reduce the 'bad' cholesterol. The oil has become the traditional fat worldwide with some of the healthiest populations. A great deal of research has been provided showing the oil is a huge plus towards the risk of heart disease because of the antioxidants and fatty acids.

You will still need to pay close attention when purchasing olive oil because it may have been extracted from the olives using chemicals or possibly diluted with other cheaper oils, such as canola and soybean. You need to be aware of refined or light olive or regular oils. The Mediterranean diet plan calls for the use of extra-virgin olive oil because it has been standardized for purity using natural methods providing the sensory qualities of its excellent taste and smell. The oil is high in phenolic antioxidants, which makes—real—olive oil beneficial.

Beverage Options: Maintaining a healthy body requires plenty of water, and the Mediterranean diet plan is not any different. Tea and coffee are allowed, but you should avoid fruit juices or sugar-sweetened beverages that contain large amounts of sugar.

White Meats: White meats are high in minerals, protein, and vitamins, but you should remove any visible fat and the skin.

Red Meats: You are allowed red meats, including lamb, pork, and beef, in small quantities. They are rich in minerals, vitamins, and protein—especially iron. Use caution because they contain more fat—specifically saturated fat—compared to the fat content found in poultry. Don't leave it out entirely; save it for a special dinner or with a stew or casserole.

Potatoes: You have noticed that potatoes are listed in the tubers group because they are a healthy choice, but it will greatly depend on how they are prepared. You receive potassium, Vitamin B, Vitamin C, and some of your daily fiber nutrients. You must consider that they contain large amounts of starch that can be quickly converted to glucose, which can be harmful and place you at risk of type 2 diabetes. Use simpler methods of cooking them, including baking, boiling, and mashing them without butter.

Desserts and Sweets: Biscuits, cakes, and sweets should be consumed in small quantities as a special treat. Not only is sugar a temptation for type 2 diabetes; it can also promote tooth decay. Many times, they may also contain higher levels of saturated fats. You can receive some nutritional value, but as a general rule—stick to small portions.

What to Eat in Moderation: Eggs, poultry, milk, butter, yogurt, and cheese

Improve the Flavor of Foods

The use of her herbs and spices provides additional flavor and aroma to your foods while on the diet plan. It will also help reduce the need for salt or fat while you're preparing your meals. Spices and herbs that adhere to a traditional Mediterranean Diet's standards include chiles, lavender, tarragon, savory, sumac, and zaatar.

These are a few more ways you can benefit from spices and herbs:

Anise Benefits: You can improve digestion as well as help reduce nausea and alleviate cramps. Prepare some anise tea after a meal to help treat indigestion and bloating gas as well as constipation.

Bay Leaf Benefits: Bay leaves contain magnesium, calcium, potassium, and Vitamins A & C. You are promoting your general health, and it is also proven to be useful in the treatment of migraines.

Basil Benefits: You can receive aid in digestion, help with gastric diseases, and help reduce flatulence. You can also protect your heart health, help reduce stress and anxiety, and help manage your diabetes. The next time you have dandruff issues, try rubbing them in your scalp after shampooing. The chemicals help eliminate dandruff and dry skin.

Black Pepper Benefits: Pepper promotes nutrient absorption in the tissues all over your body, speeds up your metabolism, and improves digestion. The main ingredient of pepper is a pipeline, which gives it a pungent taste. It can boost fat metabolism by as much as 8% for up to several hours after it's ingested. As you will see, it is used throughout your healthy Mediterranean recipes.

Cayenne Pepper Benefits: The secret ingredient in cayenne is capsaicin, a natural compound that gives fiery heat to peppers. This provides a short increase in your metabolism. The peppers are also rich in vitamins, effective as an appetite controller, smooth out digestion issues, and benefit your heart health.

Sweet & Spicy Cloves Benefits: Add cloves to hot tea for a spicy flavor. The antiseptic and germicidal ingredients in cloves will help with many types of pain including the relief of arthritis pain, gum and tooth pain, aids in digestive problems, and helps to fight infections. Use the oil of clove as an antiseptic to kill bacteria in fungal infections, itchy rashes, bruises, or burns. Just the smell of cloves can help encourage mental creativity.

Ground Chia Seeds Benefits: The seeds can absorb up to 11 times their weight in liquid. Be sure to add plenty of water and soak them for at least 5 minutes before using them in your recipes. Otherwise, you will have some uncomfortable digestion after eating them. Be sure to remain hydrated.

Cumin Benefits: The flavor of cumin and has been described as spicy, earthy, nutty, and warm. It's been long used as traditional medicine. It can help promote digestion and reduce foodborne infections. It is also beneficial for promoting weight loss and improving cholesterol and blood sugar control.

Fennel Benefits: You can receive potassium, sodium, vitamin A, calcium, vitamin C, iron, vitamin B6, and magnesium from fennel. Your bone health will show improvement with phosphate and calcium, which are excellent for your bone structure—iron and zinc or crucial for collagen production. Your heart health is also protected with vitamin C, folate, potassium, and fiber provided in the fennel.

Garlic Benefits: Garlic leads the charge of lowering your blood sugar and assisting you in weight loss. It helps control your appetite.

Ginger Benefits: Ginger is an effective diuretic that increases urine elimination. It is also known for its cholesterol-fighting properties, as a metabolism and mobility booster. Ginger also helps fight bloating issues.

Marjoram Benefits: This is used in the diet to promote healthy digestion, assist in the management of type 2 diabetes, helps to rectify hormonal imbalances, and also helps promote restful sleep and a sound mind.

Mint Benefits: Mint can be used for the treatment of nasal congestion, nausea, dizziness, and headaches. It helps to improve blood circulation, improves dental health, and helps colic in infants. Mint helps to prevent dandruff and pesky head lice.

Oregano Benefits: Oregano is very easily added to your diet and is rich in antioxidants and may also help fight bacteria. Oregano is also good for the treatment of the common cold since it helps in reducing infections, helps kill off intestinal parasites, and's also beneficial in treating menstrual cramps. One huge plus is that it also supports the body with nutrients to help support weight loss and improve digestion.

Parsley Benefits: You can help your skin, prostate, and digestive tract by making use of its high levels of a flavonoid called apigenin. It contains a powerful antioxidant and inflammatory power as well as providing remarkable anti-cancer properties.

Rosemary Benefits: The spice is known to increase hair growth, may help relieve pain, eases stress, and also helps reduce joint inflammation.

Sage Benefits: The leaves of the sage plant are also used to make medicine. It is an excellent source to improve your digestive issues, including diarrhea, stomach pain or gastritis, heartburn, and gas or flatulence. It is also beneficial for those who suffer from depression, Alzheimer's disease, memory loss, and so much more.

Tarragon Benefits: The tarragon spice is an excellent choice for maintaining your blood sugar levels, keeping your heart healthy, reduction of inflammation symptoms, improvement of digestive functions, improves central nervous system conditions, and supports healthier eyes.

Thyme Benefits: Thyme is another spice that has been used throughout history for protection from 'Black Death' as well as for embalming. (Not a pretty thought for dinner but interesting nonetheless.) It is also believed to have insecticidal and antibacterial properties. You can use it as an essential oil, as a dried herb or fresh.

As you will notice, the recipes included in your new menu plan have an extensive listing of spices. Not only do they improve your foods, but also, they improve your health at the same time!

CHAPTER 2:

Breakfast

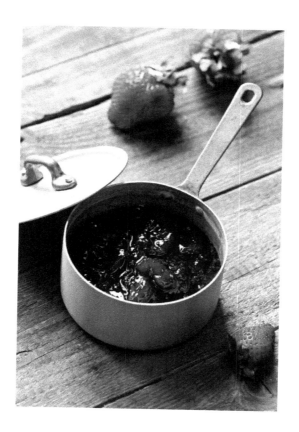

1. Mediterranean Egg Scramble

Preparation Time: 10 minutes

Cooking Time: 20 minutes

Servings: 2

Ingredients:

- 1 tbsp. of olive oil

- One yellow pepper, diced

- Two green onions, sliced

- Eight cherry tomatoes, quartered

- 2 tbsp. of black olives

- Four large eggs 1 tbsp. of capers

- ¼ tsp. of oregano, dried Ground pepper

- Fresh parsley, optional, for serving

Directions:

1. Heat oil in a frying pan. Add chopped onions and diced peppers. Cook for several minutes on medium

heat till a bit soft. Add capers, tomatoes, and olives. Cook for 1 minute more.

2. Crack eggs into the pan. Scramble promptly with a spatula or spoon. Add ground pepper and oregano. Continue to stir till eggs have cooked fully. Top with parsley, as desired. Serve while warm.

Nutrition:

Calories: 247

Protein: 13.6 g

Fat: 16.5 g

Carbohydrates: 12.8 g

2.   Avocado Green Apple Breakfast Smoothie

Preparation Time: 5 minutes

Cooking Time: 10 minutes

Servings: 2

Ingredients:

- 3 cups of spinach, fresh

- 1 Granny Smith, apple chopped

- 2 cups of coconut water

- One avocado, fresh

- One frozen banana, ripe but not soft

- 3 tbsp. of chia seeds

- 1 tsp. of honey +/- as desired

Directions:

1. Place coconut water, spinach, and apple in a food processor. Blend till smooth.

2. Add frozen banana, avocado, honey, and chia seeds. Blend till you have a creamy, smooth mixture.

3. Pour smoothie into glasses and serve while still cold.

Nutrition:

Calories: 415

Protein: 8.8 g

Fat: 21.3 g

Carbohydrates: 54.8 g

3.   Greens & Eggs Mediterranean Breakfast

Preparation Time: 10 minutes

Cooking Time: 15 minutes

Servings: 2

Ingredients:

- 1 tbsp. of olive oil

- 2 cups of rainbow chard, stemmed, chopped

- 1 cup of spinach, fresh

- ½ cup of arugula

- Four large eggs, beaten

- Two garlic cloves, minced

- ½ cup of cheddar cheese, shredded

- Kosher salt, as desired Ground pepper, as desired

Directions:

1. Heat the oil in a saucepan placed on a medium-high heat. Sauté the arugula, chard, and spinach till tender,

three minutes or so. Add the garlic. Stir while cooking till fragrant, 2 to 3 minutes.

2. Mix cheese and eggs in a medium bowl. Add to spinach mixture.

3. Cover. Cook till mixture sets, 5 to 7 minutes. Season as desired and serve.

Nutrition:

Calories: 330 Protein: 22 g

Fat: 26.7 g Carbohydrates: 4.4 g

4.   **Green on Green Smoothie**

Preparation Time: 5 minutes

Cooking Time: 0 minute

Servings: 1

Ingredients:

- 1 cup of packed baby spinach

- ½ green apple 1 tbsp. of maple syrup

- ¼ tsp. of ground cinnamon

- 1 cup of unsweetened almond milk

- ½ cup of ice

Directions:

1. In a blender, put all the prepared ingredients. Blend it until smooth. Serve.

Nutrition:

Calories: 130 Protein: 2 g

Fat: 4 g Carbohydrates: 23 g

5. Eggs with Zucchini Noodles

Preparation Time: 10 Minutes

Cooking Time: 11 Minutes

Servings: 2

Ingredients:

- Two tbsp. extra-virgin olive oil

- Three zucchinis, cut with a spiralizer

- Four eggs

- Salt and black pepper to the taste

- A pinch of red pepper flakes

- Cooking spray

- One tbsp. basil, chopped

Directions:

1. In a bowl, combine the zucchini noodles with salt, pepper, and olive oil and toss well.

2. Grease a baking sheet using cooking spray and divide the zucchini noodles into four nests on it.

3. Crash an egg on top of each nest, sprinkle salt, pepper, and pepper flakes on topmost, then bake at 350 degrees F for 11 minutes.

4. Divide the mix between plates, sprinkle the basil on top, and serve.

Nutrition:

Calories 296 Fat 23.6g

Fiber 3.3g Carbs 10.6g Protein 14.7 g

6.   Banana Oats

Preparation: 10 Minutes Cooking: 0 Minutes Servings: 2

Ingredients:

- One banana, peeled and sliced

- ¾ cup almond milk ½ cup cold-brewed coffee

- Two dates pitted

- Two tbsp. cocoa powder

- 1 cup rolled oats

- One and ½ tbsp. chia seeds

Directions:

1. In a blender, combine the banana with the milk and the rest of the ingredients, pulse, divide into bowls, and serve breakfast.

Nutrition:

Calories 451 Fat 25.1g Fiber 9.9g Carbs 55.4 gProtein 9.3g

7.   Veggie Bowls

Preparation Time: 10 Minutes

Cooking Time: 5 Minutes

Servings: 4

Ingredients:

- One tbsp. olive oil

- 1-pound asparagus, trimmed and roughly chopped

- 3 cups kale, shredded

- 3 cups Brussels sprouts, shredded

- ½ cup hummus

- One avocado, peeled, pitted, and sliced

- Four eggs, soft boiled, peeled and sliced

For the dressing:

- Two tbsp. lemon juice

- One garlic clove, minced

- Two tsp. Dijon mustard

- Two tbsp. olive oil

- Salt and black pepper to the taste

Directions:

1. Heat a pan put two tablespoon of oil over medium-high heat, then add the asparagus and sauté for 5 minutes, stirring often.

2. In a bowl, combine the other two tbsp. oil with the lemon juice, garlic, mustard, salt, and pepper and whisk well.

3. In a salad bowl, combine the asparagus with the kale, sprouts, hummus, avocado, and eggs and toss gently.

4. Add the dressing, toss, and serve for breakfast.

Nutrition:

Calories 323 Fat 21g

Fiber 10.9g

Carbs 24.8g

8.   Avocado and Apple Smoothie

Preparation: 5 Minutes Cooking: 0 Minutes Servings: 2

Ingredients:

- 3 cups spinach

- One green apple, cored and chopped

- One avocado, peeled, pitted, and chopped

- Three tbsp. chia seeds One tsp. honey

- One banana, frozen and peeled

- 2 cups of coconut water

Directions:

1. In your blender, blend the spinach with the apple and the rest of the ingredients. Pulse and divide into glasses and serve.

Nutrition:

Calories 168 Fat 10.1 g Fiber 6g Carbs 21g Protein 2.1g

CHAPTER 3:

Main Dishes

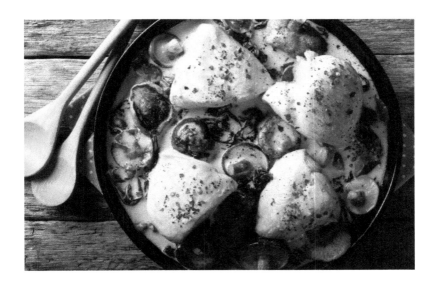

9.   Zoodles with Walnut Pesto

Preparation Time: 10 minutes

Cooking Time: 10 minutes Serving: 4

Ingredients

- Four medium zucchinis, spiralized

- ¼ cup extra-virgin olive oil, divided

- 1 tsp. minced garlic, divided

- ½ tsp. crushed red pepper

- ¼ tsp. freshly ground black pepper, divided

- ¼ tsp. kosher salt, divided

- 2 tbsp. grated Parmesan cheese, divided

- 1 cup packed fresh basil leaves

- ¾ cup walnut pieces, divided

Directions

1. In a large bowl, stir together the zoodles, 1 tbsp. of the olive oil, ½ tsp. of the minced garlic, red pepper,

1/8 tsp. of the black pepper, and 1/8 tsp. of the salt. Set aside.

2. Heat ½ tbsp. of the oil in a large skillet over medium-high heat. Add half of the zoodles to the skillet and cook for 5 minutes, stirring constantly. Transfer the cooked zoodles into a bowl. Repeat with another ½ tbsp. of the oil and the remaining zoodles. When done, add the cooked zoodles to the bowl.

3. Make the pesto: Prepared the food processor, combine the remaining ½ tsp. of the minced garlic, 1/8 tsp. of the black pepper, and 1/8 tsp. of the salt, 1 tbsp. of the Parmesan, basil leaves, and ¼ cup of the walnuts. Pulse until smooth and then slowly drizzle the remaining 2 tbsp. of the oil into the pesto. Pulse again until well combined.

4. Add the pesto to the zoodles along with the remaining 1 tbsp. of the Parmesan and the remaining ½ cup of the walnuts. Toss to coat well.

5. Serve immediately.

Nutrition

Calories: 166

Fat: 16.0g

Protein: 4.0g

Carbs: 3.0g

Fiber: 2.0g

Sodium: 307mg

10.   Cheesy Sweet Potato Burgers

Preparation Time: 10 minutes

Cooking Time: 20 minutes

Serving: 4

Ingredients

- One large sweet potato (about 8 ounces / 227 g)

- 2 tbsp. extra-virgin olive oil, divided

- 1 cup chopped onion

- One large egg One garlic clove

- 1 cup old-fashioned rolled oats

- 1 tbsp. dried oregano

- 1 tbsp. balsamic vinegar ¼ tsp. kosher salt

- ½ cup crumbled Gorgonzola cheese

Directions

1. Make puncture to the sweet potato all over using a fork, and microwave on high for 4 to 5 minutes, until

softened in the center. Cool slightly before slicing in half.

2. Meanwhile, in a large skillet over medium-high heat, heat 1 tbsp. of the olive oil. Stir in the onion and sauté for five minutes.

3. Spoon the flesh of a sweet potato out of the skin and put the meat in a food processor. Add the cooked onion, egg, garlic, oats, oregano, vinegar, and salt. Pulse until smooth. Add the cheese and pulse four times to barely combine.

4. Form the mixture into four burgers. Place the burgers on a plate, and press to flatten each to about ¾-inch thick.

5. Wipe out the skillet use a paper towel. Heat the remaining 1 tbsp. of the oil over medium-high heat for about 2 minutes. Add the burgers to the hot oil

then reduce the heat to medium—Cook the burgers for 5 minutes per side.

6. Move the burgers to a plate and serve.

Nutrition

Calories: 290 Fat: 12.0g

Protein: 12.0g

Carbs: 43.0g

Fiber: 8.0g

Sodium: 566mg

11.   Eggplant and Zucchini Gratin

Preparation Time: 10 minutes

Cooking Time: 19 minutes

Serving: 6

Ingredients

- Two large zucchinis, finely chopped

- One large eggplant, finely chopped

- ¼ tsp. kosher salt

- ¼ tsp. freshly ground black pepper

- 3 tbsp. extra-virgin olive oil, divided

- ¾ cup unsweetened almond milk

- 1 tbsp. all-purpose flour

- ¹/3 cup plus 2 tbsp. grated Parmesan cheese, divided

- 1 cup chopped tomato

- 1 cup diced fresh Mozzarella

- ¼ cup fresh basil leaves

Directions

1. Preheat the oven and set to 425°F (220°C).

2. In a large bowl, toss together the zucchini, eggplant, salt, and pepper.

3. In a prepared large skillet over medium-high heat, heat 1 tbsp. of the oil. Add half of the veggie mixture to the skillet. Stir for a few times, then cover and cook for about 4 minutes, stirring occasionally. Pour the cooked veggies into a baking dish. Place the skillet back on the heat, add 1 tbsp. of the oil and repeat with the remaining veggies. Add the veggies to the baking dish.

4. For the meantime, heat the milk in the microwave for 1 minute. Set aside.

5. Place a medium saucepan over medium heat. Add the remaining 1 tbsp. of the oil and flour to the saucepan. Whisk together until well blended.

6. Slowly pour the warm milk into the saucepan, whisking the entire time. Continue to whisk frequently until the mixture thickens a bit. Add $1/3$ cup of the Parmesan cheese and whisk until melted. Pour the cheese sauce over the vegetables in the baking dish and mix well.

7. Fold in the tomatoes and Mozzarella cheese—roast in the oven for 10 minutes, or until the gratin is almost set and not runny.

8. Top with the fresh basil leaves and the remaining 2 tbsp. of the Parmesan cheese before serving.

Nutrition

Calories: 122 Fat: 5.0g Protein: 10.0g

Carbs: 11.0g

Fiber: 4.0g

Sodium: 364mg

12.   Veggie-Stuffed Portobello Mushrooms

Preparation Time: 5 minutes

Cooking Time: 24-25 minutes

Serving: 6

Ingredients

- 3 tbsp. extra-virgin olive oil, divided

- 1 cup diced onion

- Two garlic cloves, minced

- One large zucchini, diced

- 3 cups chopped mushrooms

- 1 cup chopped tomato

- 1 tsp. dried oregano

- ¼ tsp. kosher salt

- ¼ tsp. crushed red pepper

- Six large portobello mushrooms, stems, and gills removed

- Cooking spray

- 4 ounces (113 g) fresh mozzarella cheese, shredded

Directions

1. In a large skillet over medium heat, heat 2 tbsp. of the oil. Add the onion and sauté for 4 minutes. Stir in the garlic and sauté for 1 minute.

2. Stir in the zucchini, mushrooms, tomato, oregano, salt, and red pepper. Cook for 10 minutes, stirring constantly. Remove from the heat.

3. Meanwhile, Set the grill and heat a grill pan over medium-high heat.

4. Brush the remaining 1 tbsp. of the oil over the portobello mushroom caps. Place the mushrooms, bottom-side down, on the grill pan. Cover with a sheet of aluminum foil sprayed with nonstick cooking spray—Cook for 5 minutes.

5. Flip the mushroom caps over, and spoon about ½ cup of the cooked vegetable mixture into each cap. Top each with about 2½ tbsp. of the Mozzarella.

6. Cover and then grill for 4 to 5 minutes, or until the cheese is melted.

7. Using a spatula, transfer the portobello mushrooms to a plate. Let cool for about 5 minutes before serving.

Nutrition

Calories: 111

Fat: 4.0g

Protein: 11.0g

Carbs: 11.0g

Fiber: 4.0g

Sodium: 314mg

13.   Brussels sprouts Linguine

Preparation: 5 minutes Cooking: 25 minutes Serving: 4

Ingredients

- 8 ounces (227 g) whole-wheat linguine

- $1/3$ cup plus 2 tbsp. extra-virgin olive oil, divided

- One medium sweet onion, diced

- 2 to 3 garlic cloves, smashed

- 8 ounces (227 g) Brussels sprouts, chopped

- ½ cup chicken stock $1/3$ cup dry white wine

- ½ cup shredded Parmesan cheese

- One lemon, quartered

Directions

1. Bring a large pot of water let it boil and cook the pasta for about 5 minutes, or until al dente. Drain the pasta and reserve 1 cup of the pasta water. Mix the cooked pasta with 2 tbsp. of the olive oil. Set aside.

2. In a large skillet, heat the remaining ¹/3 cup of the olive oil over medium heat. Add the onion to the skillet then sauté for about 4 minutes, or until tender. Add the smashed garlic cloves and sauté for 1 minute, or until fragrant.

3. Stir in the Brussels sprouts and cook covered for 10 minutes. Pour in the chicken stock to prevent burning. Once the Brussels sprouts have wilted and are fork-tender, add white wine and cook for about 5 minutes, or until reduced.

4. Add the pasta to the skillet and add the pasta water as needed.

5. Top with the Parmesan cheese and squeeze the lemon over the dish right before eating.

Nutrition

Calories: 502 Fat: 31.0g Protein: 15.0g Carbs: 50.0g

Fiber: 9.0g Sodium: 246mg

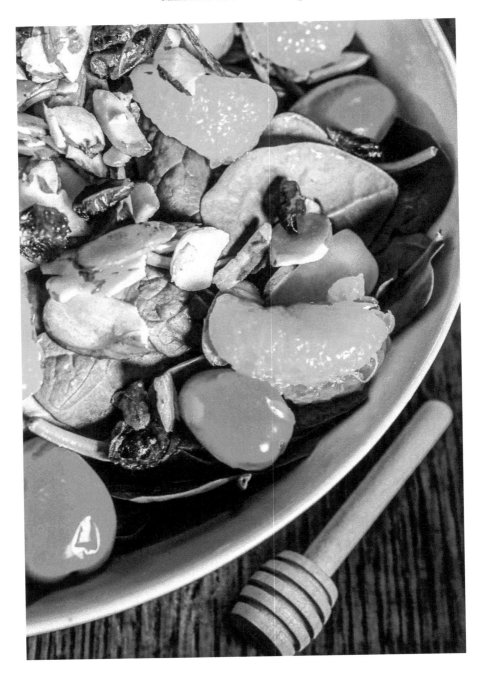

CHAPTER 4:

Side and Salad Recipes

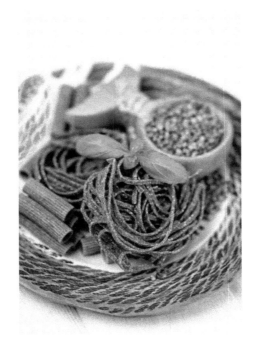

14.   Asparagus Couscous

Preparation Time: 15 minutes

Cooking Time: 30 Minutes

Servings: 6

Ingredients:

- 1 cup Goat Cheese, Garlic & Herb Flavored

- 1 ½ lbs. Asparagus, Trimmed & Chopped into 1 Inch Pieces

- 1 tbsp. Olive Oil 1 Clove Garlic, Minced

- ¼ tsp. Black Pepper One ¾ Cup Water

- 8 Oz. Whole Wheat Couscous, Uncooked

- ¼ tsp. Sea Salt, Fine

Directions:

1. Preheat your oven set at 425°F, and then put your goat cheese on the counter. It needs to come to room temperature.

2. Get out a bowl and mix your oil, pepper, garlic, and asparagus. Spread the asparagus on a baking sheet and roast for ten minutes. Make sure to stir at least once.

3. Remove it from the pan, and place your asparagus in a serving bowl.

4. Get out a medium saucepan, and bring your water to a boil. Add in your salt and couscous. Reduce the heat to medium-low, and then cover your saucepan. Cook for twelve minutes. All your water should be absorbed.

5. Pour the couscous in a bowl with asparagus, and ad din your goat cheese. Stir until melted, and serve warm.

Nutrition:

Calories: 263 Protein: 11 g

Fat: 9 g Carbs: 36 g

15. Easy Spaghetti Squash

Preparation Time: 15 minutes

Cooking Time: 25 Minutes

Servings: 4

Ingredients:

- 2 Spring Onions, Chopped Fine

- 3 Cloves Garlic, Minced

- 1 Zucchini, Diced1 Red Bell Pepper, Diced

- 1 tbsp. Italian Seasoning

- 1 Tomato, Small & Chopped Fine

- 1 tbsp. Parsley, Fresh & Chopped

- Pinch Lemon Pepper

- Dash Sea Salt, Fine

- 4 Oz. Feta Cheese, Crumbled

- 3 Italian Sausage Links, Casing Removed

- 2 tbsp. Olive Oil

- 1 Spaghetti Sauce, Halved Lengthwise

Directions:

1. Preheat your oven set at 350°F, and get out a large baking sheet. Coat it with cooking spray, and then put your squash on it with the cut side down.

2. Bake at 350°F for forty-five minutes. It should be tender.

3. Turn the squash over, and bake for five more minutes. Scrape the strands into a larger bowl.

4. Heat a tbsp. of olive oil in a skillet, and then add in your Italian sausage—Cook at eight minutes before removing it and placing it in a bowl.

5. Add another tbsp. of olive oil to the skillet and cook your garlic and onions until softened. That will take five minutes.

6. Throw in your Italian seasoning, red peppers, and zucchini. Cook for another five minutes. Your vegetables should be softened.

7. Mix in your feta cheese and squash, cooking until the cheese has melted.

8. Stir in your sausage, and then season with lemon pepper and salt. Serve with parsley and tomato.

Nutrition:

Calories: 423

Protein: 18 g

Fat: 30 g

Carbs: 22 g

16.   Garbanzo Bean Salad

Preparation Time: 10 minutes

Cooking Time: 0 minutes

Servings: 4

Ingredients:

- One and ½ cups cucumber, cubed

- 15 oz. canned garbanzo beans drained and rinsed

- 3 oz. black olives, pitted and sliced

- One tomato, chopped

- ¼ cup red onion, chopped

- 5 cups salad greens

- A pinch of salt and black pepper

- ½ cup feta cheese, crumbled

- 3 tbsp. olive oil

- 1 tbsp. lemon juice

- ¼ cup parsley, chopped

Directions:

1. In a salad bowl, combine the garbanzo beans with the cucumber, tomato, and the rest of the ingredients except the cheese and toss.

2. Divide the mix into small bowls, sprinkle the cheese on top, and serve for breakfast.

Nutrition:

Calories 268

Fat 16.5 g

Fiber 7.6 g

Carbs 36.6 g

Protein 9.4 g

17.   Spiced Chickpeas Bowls

Preparation Time: 10 minutes

Cooking Time: 30 minutes

Servings: 4

Ingredients:

- 15 oz. canned chickpeas drained and rinsed

- ¼ tsp. cardamom, ground

- ½ tsp. cinnamon powder

- One and ½ tsp. turmeric powder

- 1 tsp. coriander, ground

- 1 tbsp. olive oil

- A pinch of salt and black pepper

- ¾ cup Greek yogurt

- ½ cup green olives pitted and halved

- ½ cup cherry tomatoes halved

- One cucumber, sliced

Directions:

1. On a lined baking sheet, spread the chickpeas, add the cardamom, cinnamon, turmeric, coriander, the oil, salt, and pepper, toss and bake at 375°F for 30 minutes.

2. In a bowl, combine the roasted chickpeas with the rest of the ingredients, toss, and serve breakfast.

Nutrition:

Calories 519

Fat 34.5 g

Fiber 13.6 g

Carbs 36.6 g

Protein 11.4 g

18. Balsamic Asparagus

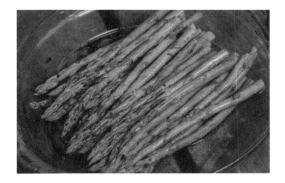

Preparation time: 10 minutes

Cooking time: 15 minutes Servings: 4

Ingredients:

- 3 tbsp. olive oil Three garlic cloves, minced

- 2 tbsp. shallot, chopped

- Salt and black pepper to the taste

- 2 tsp. balsamic vinegar

- One and ½ pound asparagus, trimmed

Directions:

1. Heat a pan with the oil over medium-high heat, add the garlic and the shallot and sauté for 3 minutes.

2. Add the rest of the ingredients, cook for 12 minutes more, divide between plates and serve as a side dish.

Nutrition:

Calories 100

Fat: 10.5 g

Fiber: 1.2 g

Carbs: 2.3 g

Protein: 2.1 g

19. Lime Cucumber Mix

Preparation: 10 minutes Cooking: 0 minutes   Servings: 8

Ingredients:

- Four cucumbers, chopped

- ½ cup green bell pepper, chopped

- One yellow onion, chopped One chili pepper, chopped One garlic clove, minced 1 tsp. parsley, chopped 2 tbsp. lime juice 1 tbsp. dill, chopped

- Salt and black pepper to the taste

- 1 tbsp. olive oil

Directions:

1. In a prepared large bowl, mix the cucumber with the bell peppers and the rest of the ingredients, toss and serve as a side dish.

Nutrition:

Calories 123 Fat 4.3 g Fiber 2.3g Carbs 5.6g Protein 2 g

20.   Walnuts Cucumber Mix

Preparation: 5 minutes Cooking: 0 minutes Servings: 2

Ingredients:

- Two cucumbers, chopped 1 tbsp. olive oil

- Salt and black pepper to the taste

- One red chili pepper, dried 1 tbsp. lemon juice

- 3 tbsp. walnuts, chopped

- 1 tbsp. balsamic vinegar

- 1 tsp. chives, chopped

Directions:

1. In a prepared bowl, mix the cucumbers with the oil and the rest of the ingredients, toss and serve as a side dish.

Nutrition:

Calories 121 Fat 2.3g Fiber 2.0g Carbs 6.7g Protein 2.4

21. Cheesy Beet Salad

Preparation time: 10 minutes

Cooking time: 1 hour

Servings: 4

Ingredients:

- Four beets, peeled and cut into wedges

- 3 tbsp. olive oil

- Salt and black pepper to the taste

- ¼ cup lime juice

- Eight slices goat cheese, crumbled

- 1/3 cup walnuts, chopped

- 1 tbsp. chives, chopped

Directions:

1. In a roasting pan, combine the beets with the oil, salt, and pepper, toss and bake at 400 degrees F for 1 hour.

2. Cool the beets down, transfer them to a bowl, add the rest of the ingredients, toss and serve as a side salad.

Nutrition:

Calories: 156 Fat 4.2g

Fiber 3.4g Carbs 6.5g Protein 4 g

CHAPTER 5:

Seafood

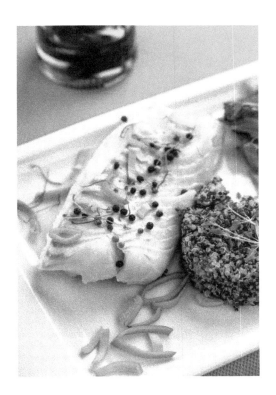

22.   Grilled Sardines

Preparation Time: 5 minutes

Cooking Time: 15 minutes

Servings: 4

Ingredients:

- 3 Tbsps. Of Vegetable Oil.

- ¾ Tsp. Of Pepper.

- 11/2 Tsp. Of Dried Oregano.

- 3 Tbsps. Of Lemon Juice.

- ½ Cup of Extra-Virgin Olive Oil (Divided).

- 2 Tsp. Of Salt.

- Clean Gutted and Scaled 2 Pounds of Fresh Sardine (the Head Removed)

Directions:

1. Preheat your set to a medium-high heat.

2. Rinse the sardine and pat it dry with a paper towel, then brush with olive oil on both sides. Sprinkle with pepper and salt on both sides.

3. Wipe the grill surface with oil. Place each sardine on the grill and grill for 2-3 minutes; while grilling, drizzle the sardine with olive oil and lemon juice.

4. Sprinkle with oregano and serve.

Nutrition:

Calories: 231

Carb: 0.6g

Protein: 26g

Fat: 13.6g

23.   Halibut Roulade

Preparation: 5 minutes Cooking: 10 minutes Servings: 6

Ingredients:

- 1lbs of Halibut Fillet.

- ½ Pound Shrimp.   3 Limes.

- ½ Bunch Cilantro.

- 3 Cloves Garlic.   ½ Leeks.

- 1 tbsp. Of Olive Oil.

- Freshly-Cracked Black Pepper.

- 1 Cup of Seafood Demi-Glace Reduction Sauce.

Directions:

1. Before starting, soak 12 wooden skewers in water for a minimum of 2 hours. Preheat the grill.

2. For the fillet, wash and chill, remove the shell and tail of the shrimp. Slice the shrimp in half along the length and remove the vein.

3. Squeeze two limes for juice and cut one into wedges. Grate the rind for zest.

4. Reserve some cilantro and chop the remaining ones. Slice the leek and mince the garlic.

5. Cut the halibut fillet across the length to about ½-3/4 inch thick. Spread and layer with shrimp, zest, cilantro, leek, and garlic, and carefully roll-up.

6. Cut the fillet into six pinwheels and insert two skewers into each pinwheel, forming X. brush with oil and grill for 4minutes per side or until it is golden brown.

7. Drizzle with oil and garnish with the remaining cilantro, zest, ½ tsp. of pepper. Serve with demi-glace reduction sauce.

Nutrition:

Calories: 342 Carb: 11g Protein: 46g

24. Glazed Broiled Salmon

Preparation Time: 20 minutes

Cooking Time: 20 minutes

Servings: 4-6

Ingredients:

Glaze:

- 2 Tbsp. Dark Brown Sugar.

- 4 Tsp. Dijon Mustard.

- 1 Tbsp. Soy Sauce.

- 1 Tsp. Rice Vinegar.

Salmon:

- 2 Medium Size Salmon Fillets.

Directions:

1. Preheat oven to broil.

2. Mix glaze ingredients.

3. Clean and de-bone salmon.

4. Coat with glaze the side of the salmon. Place on a baking sheet.

5. Broil salmon within 8-10 inches of the coils, be careful not to get too close; you don't want it cooking too fast.

6. It is done when it opaque and flakes easily in the center.

Nutrition:

Calories: 10 Carb: 0.86g

Protein: 0.31g Fat: 0.59g

25. Honey-Mustard Roasted Salmon

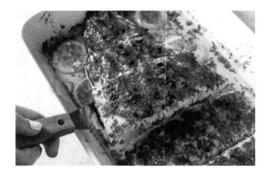

Preparation Time: 5 minutes

Cooking Time: 25 minutes

Servings: 6

Ingredients:

- Cooking Spray.

- 1 Lemon Sliced.

- 1 (3-Lb.) Salmon Fillet.

- Kosher Salt.

- Freshly Ground Black Pepper.

- 1/2 C. Whole Grain Mustard.

- 1/4 C. Extra-Virgin Olive Oil.

- 1/4 C. Honey.

- 2 Cloves Garlic, Minced.

- 1/2 Tsp. Red Pepper Flakes.

Directions:

1. Freshly chopped parsley for serving.

2. Preheat oven set to 400° and grease a 9"-x-13" baking dish with cooking spray. Place lemon slices on the bottom of the dish and place salmon on top. Put seasoning with salt and pepper.

3. In a medium bowl, whisk together mustard, oil, honey, garlic, and red pepper flakes. Put seasonings with salt and pepper, then pour the sauce over salmon.

4. Roast salmon until cooked through and flakes easily with a fork, 20 minutes.

5. Turn oven to broil and broil another 5 minutes, if desired.

6. Garnish with parsley before serving.

Nutrition:

Calories: 115 Carb: 19.74g

Protein: 1.49g   Fat: 4.14g

26. Asian-Inspired Tuna Lettuce Wraps

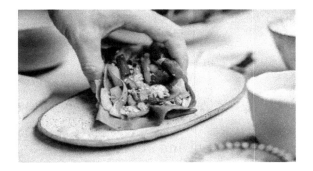

Preparation Time: 30 minutes

Cooking Time: 0 minutes

Servings: 6-7

Ingredients:

For the wraps:

- 1 Head Butter Lettuce or Romaine Lettuce

- 3 Packets Good Catch Foods Tuna

- 1 Large Carrot, Peeled into Ribbons

- 1 Large Red Pepper, Sliced

- 1/4 cup Green Onions, Roughly Chopped

- A Handful of Fresh Cilantro

For the sauce:

- 1 Tbsp. Fresh Ginger, Grated

- 2 Cloves of Garlic, Grated

- 1 1/2 Tbsp. Soy Sauce or Coconut Aminos

- 2 Tbsp. Sesame Oil and Seeds

- Juice of Half A Lime

- 1 Tbsp. Rice Wine Vinegar

- 2 Tbsp. Vegetable Oil

- 2 Tbsp. Maple Syrup

Directions:

1. To a prepared medium-sized bowl, add your Good Catch Foods Tuna and all your sauce ingredients. Mash up the stir gently using a fork and mix it well. Set aside to marry for 15 minutes until your lettuce wraps are assembled.

2. While you wait, prepare all your choice of vegetables and set them aside.

3. If you like to add 2-3 pieces of butter lettuce or one piece of Romaine as the base to create your lettuce wraps, then begin filling with veggies + tuna!

4. Enjoy like you would at taco (butter lettuce) or pizza (romaine lettuce).

Nutrition:

Calories: 81

Carb: 7.52g

Protein: 1.18g

Fat: 5.42g

27.   Mediterranean Grilled Sea Bass

Preparation Time: 10 minutes

Cooking Time: 12 minutes

Servings: 4

Ingredients:

- Two lemons

- 3 tbsp. olive oil

- 1 tbsp. chopped fresh oregano leaves

- 1 tsp. ground coriander

- 1 1/4 tsp. salt

- Two whole sea bass, cleaned and scaled (about 1 1/2 lbs. each)

- 1/4 tsp. ground black pepper

- Two large oregano sprigs

Directions:

1. Preheat gas grill over medium heat.

2. For the meantime, from 1 lemon, grate 1 tbsp. peel and squeeze 2 tbsp. juice. Cut half of the remaining lemon into slices, the other half into wedges. In a small bowl, stir lemon juice and peel, oil, chopped oregano, coriander, and 1/4 tsp. salt.

3. Rinse fish and pat dry use paper towels. Make three slashes on both sides of each fish. Sprinkle inside and out with pepper and the remaining 1 tsp. salt. Put lemon slices and oregano sprigs inside fish cavities. Place fish in a 13" by 9" glass baking dish. Rub half of the oil mixture over the fish's outsides; reserve the remaining oil mixture for drizzling overcooked fish. Let rest at room temperature for 15 minutes.

4. Lightly grease grill rack; place fish on hot rack. Cover grill and cook fish for 12 to 14 minutes or until fish just turns opaque throughout and thickest part flakes easily when tested with a fork, turning fish over once.

5. To serve, place fish on the cutting board. Working with one fish at a time, with a knife, cut along backbone from head to tail. Slide wide metal spatula or cake server under the top fillet's front section and lift off from backbone; transfer to a platter. Gently pull-out backbone and rib bones from bottom fillet and discard. Transfer bottom fillet to platter. Repeat with the second fish—drizzle fillets with the remaining oil mixture. Serve with lemon wedges.

Nutrition:

Calories305

Protein: 40g

Carbohydrate: 1g

Fat: 15g

Fiber: 0g

CHAPTER 6:

Poultry

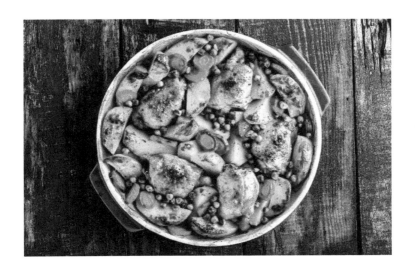

28.   Chicken and Black Beans

Preparation Time: 10 minutes

Cooking Time: 20 minutes

Serving: 4

Servings: 4

Cooking Time: 20 Minutes

Ingredients:

- 12 oz. chicken breast, skinless, boneless, chopped

- 1 tbsp. taco seasoning

- 1 tbsp. nut oil

- ½ tsp. cayenne pepper

- ½ tsp. salt

- ½ tsp. garlic, chopped

- ½ red onion, sliced

- 1/3 cup black beans, canned, rinsed

- ½ cup Mozzarella, shredded

Directions:

1. Rub the chopped chicken breast with taco seasoning, salt, and cayenne pepper.

2. Place the chicken in the skillet, add nut oil and roast it for 10 minutes over medium heat. Mix up the chicken pieces from time to time to avoid burning.

3. After this, transfer the chicken to the plate.

4. Add sliced onion and then garlic to the skillet. Roast the vegetables for 5 minutes. Stir them constantly. Then add black beans and stir well—Cook the ingredients for 2 minutes more.

5. Add the chopped chicken and mix up well. Top the meal with Mozzarella cheese.

6. Close the lid and cook the meal for 3 minutes.

Nutrition:

Calories 209 Fat 6.4 Fiber 2.8 Carbs 13.7, 22.7

29.   Coconut Chicken

Preparation Time: 10 minutes

Cooking Time: 5 minutes

Serving: 4

Ingredients:

- 6 oz. chicken fillet

- ¼ cup of sparkling water

- One egg

- 3 tbsp. coconut flakes

- 1 tbsp. coconut oil

- 1 tsp. Greek Seasoning

Directions:

1. Cut the chicken fillet into small pieces (nuggets).

2. Then crack the egg in the bowl and whisk it.

3. Mix up together egg and sparkling water.

4. Add Greek seasoning and stir gently.

5. Dip the chicken nuggets in the egg mixture and then coat in the coconut flakes.

6. Melt the coconut oil in the skillet and heat it until it is shimmering.

7. Then add prepared chicken nuggets.

8. Roast them for 1 minute from each or until they are light brown.

9. Dry the cooked chicken nuggets with the paper towels help and transfer them to the serving plates.

Nutrition:

Calories 141 Fat 8.9

Fiber 0.3 Carbs 1 Protein 13.9

30. Ginger Chicken Drumsticks

Preparation Time: 10 minutes

Cooking Time: 30 minutes

Serving: 4

Ingredients:

- Four chicken drumsticks

- One apple, grated

- 1 tbsp. curry paste

- 4 tbsp. milk

- 1 tsp. coconut oil

- 1 tsp. chili flakes

- ½ tsp. minced ginger

Directions:

1. Mix up together grated apple, curry paste, milk, chili flakes, and minced garlic.

2. Put coconut oil in the skillet and melt it.

3. Add apple mixture and stir well.

4. Then add chicken drumsticks and mix up well.

5. Roast the chicken for 2 minutes from each side.

6. Then preheat the oven to 360F.

7. Place the skillet with chicken drumsticks in the oven and bake for 25 minutes.

Nutrition:

Calories 150

Fat 6.4g

Fiber 1.4g

Carbs 9.7g

Protein 13.5 g

31.   Parmesan Chicken

Preparation Time: 10 minutes

Cooking Time: 30 minutes

Serving: 3

Ingredients:

- 1-pound chicken breast, skinless, boneless

- 2 oz. Parmesan, grated

- 1 tsp. dried oregano

- ½ tsp. dried cilantro

- 1 tbsp. Panko bread crumbs

- One egg, beaten

- 1 tsp. turmeric

Directions:

1. Cut the chicken breast into three servings.

2. Then combine Parmesan, oregano, cilantro, bread crumbs, and turmeric.

3. Dip the chicken servings in the beaten egg carefully.

4. Then coat every chicken piece in the cheese-bread crumbs mixture.

5. Line the baking tray using the baking paper.

6. Arrange the chicken pieces in the tray.

7. Bake the chicken for 30 minutes at 365F.

Nutrition:

Calories 267 Fat 9.5

Fiber 0.5 Carbs 3.2 Protein 40.4

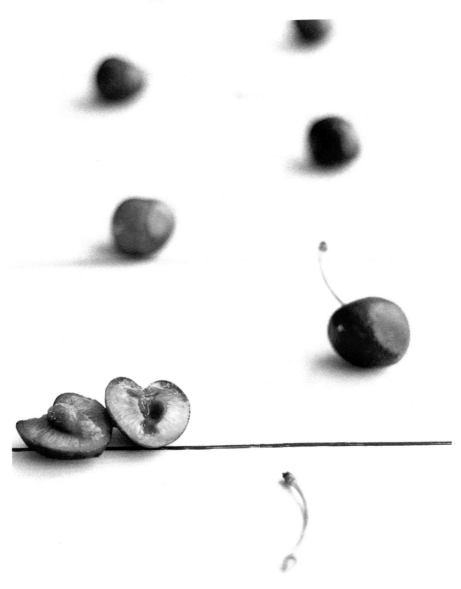

CHAPTER 7:

Snack and Appetizer

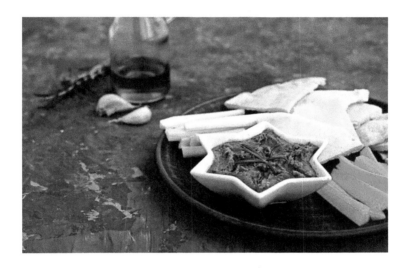

32. Cucumber Sandwich Bites

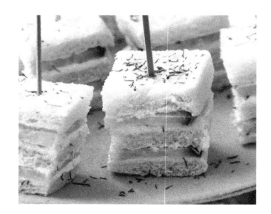

Preparation Time: 5 minutes

Cooking Time: 0 minutes

Servings: 12

Ingredients:

- One cucumber, sliced

- Eight slices of whole wheat bread

- 2 tbsp. cream cheese, soft

- 1 tbsp. chives, chopped

- ¼ cup avocado, peeled, pitted, and mashed

- 1 tsp. mustard

- Salt and black pepper to the taste

Directions:

1. Spread the mashed avocado on each bread slice, also spread the rest of the ingredients except the cucumber slices.

2. Divide the cucumber slices into the bread slices, cut each piece in thirds, arrange on a platter and serve as an appetizer.

Nutrition:

Calories 187 Fat 12.4 g

Fiber 2.1 g Carbs 4.5 g Protein 8.2 g

33. Cucumber Rolls

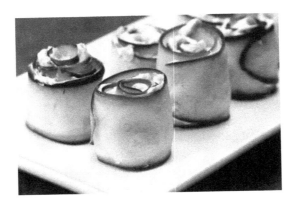

Preparation Time: 5 minutes

Cooking Time: 0 minutes

Servings: 6

Ingredients:

- One big cucumber, sliced lengthwise

- 1 tbsp. parsley, chopped

- 8 ounces canned tuna, drained and mashed

- Salt and black pepper to the taste   1 tsp. lime juice

Directions:

1. Arrange cucumber slices on a working surface, divide the rest of the ingredients, and roll.

2. Arrange all the rolls on a platter and serve as an appetizer.

Nutrition:

Calories 200

Fat 6 g

Fiber 3.4 g

Carbs 7.6 g

Protein 3.5 g

34. Olives and Cheese Stuffed Tomatoes

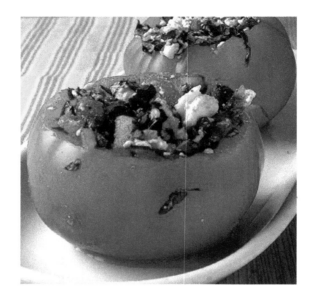

Preparation Time: 10 minutes

Cooking Time: 0 minutes

Servings: 24

Ingredients:

- 24 cherry tomatoes, top cut off, and insides scooped out

- 2 tbsp. olive oil

- ¼ tsp. red pepper flakes

- ½ cup feta cheese, crumbled

- 2 tbsp. black olive paste

- ¼ cup mint, torn

Directions:

1. In a bowl, mix the olives paste with the rest of the ingredients except the cherry tomatoes and whisk.

2. Stuff the cherry tomatoes with this mix, arrange them all on a platter, and serve as an appetizer.

Nutrition:

Calories 136; Fat 8.6 g

Fiber 4.8 g Carbs 5.6 g Protein 5.1 g

35.   Tomato Salsa

Preparation Time: 5 minutes   Cooking Time: 0 minutes

Servings: 6

Ingredients:

- One garlic clove, minced

- 4 tbsp. olive oil

- Five tomatoes, cubed

- 1 tbsp. balsamic vinegar

- ¼ cup basil, chopped

- 1 tbsp. parsley, chopped

- 1 tbsp. chives, chopped

- Salt and black pepper to the taste

- Pita chips for serving

Directions:

1. In a prepared bowl, mix the tomatoes with the garlic and the rest of the ingredients except the pita chips,

stir, divide into small cups and serve with the pita chips on the side.

Nutrition:

Calories 160 Fat 13.7 g

Fiber 5.5 g Carbs 10.1 g Protein 2.2 g

36.   Chili Mango and Watermelon Salsa

Preparation: 5 minutes Cooking: 0 minutes Servings: 12

Ingredients:

- One red tomato, chopped

- Salt and black pepper to the taste

- 1 cup watermelon, seedless, peeled, and cubed

- One red onion, chopped

- Two mangos, peeled and chopped

- Two chili peppers, chopped

- ¼ cup cilantro, chopped

- 3 tbsp. lime juice

- Pita chips for serving

Directions:

1. In a bowl, mix the tomato with the watermelon, the onion, and the rest of the ingredients except the pita chips and toss well.

2. Divide the mix into small cups and serve with pita chips on the side.

Nutrition:

Calories 62 Fat 4g

Fiber 1.3 g Carbs 3.9 g

Protein 2.3 g

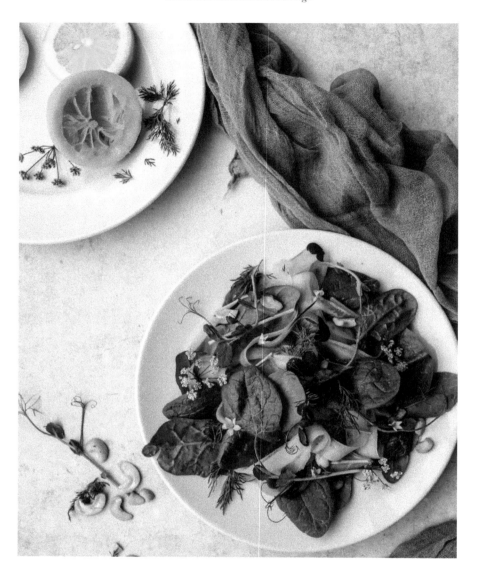

CHAPTER 8:

Meat

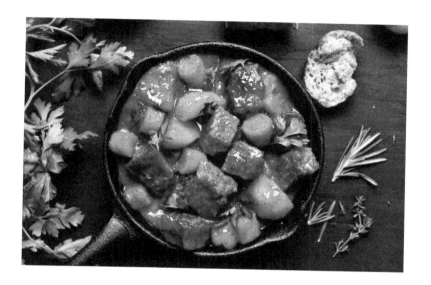

37.   Moroccan Beef Koftas

Preparation Time: 5 minutes

Cooking Time: 13 minutes

Servings: 2

Ingredients:

- 1/2 pound ground beef

- One small red onion, finely chopped

- 1 tsp. garlic, minced

- 1 tbsp. olive oil

- Sea salt to taste

- Ground black pepper, to taste

- 1/4 tsp. ground coriander

- 1/2 tsp. paprika

- 1/2 tsp. turmeric

- 1/4 tsp. ground cumin

- 1/4 tsp. allspice

Directions

1. Combine thoroughly all ingredients in a mixing bowl.

2. Shape the meat into two thick sausages and thread a bamboo skewer through each sausage.

3. Preheat your grill for medium-high heat. Lower the koftas onto a lightly oiled grill. Grill for about 13 minutes, turning them over once or twice to promote even cooking.

4. An instant-read thermometer should read160 degrees F. Serve with lemon slices or cold plain yogurt if desired. Bon appétit!

Nutrition:

Calories: 308 Fat: 21.4g

Carbs: 6.9g Protein: 23.1g

38. Beef Tenderloin Salad

Preparation Time: 10 minutes

Cooking Time: 10 minutes

Servings: 4

Ingredients

- 2 tbsp. olive oil 1 pound beef tenderloin, sliced

- Sea salt to taste

- Ground black pepper, to taste

- 1/2 tsp. paprika

- 1 tsp. oregano

- One red onion, sliced

- 2 Roma tomatoes, sliced

- 1 Persian cucumber, sliced

- 2 cups Romaine lettuce, torn into pieces

- 2 tbsp. red wine vinegar

- One avocado, peeled and sliced

- 4 ounces canned cannellini beans, drained

- 1 (6 ½-inch) pita, cut into wedges and toasted

Directions

1. Pat dries the beef tenderloin with paper towels. Season the meat with salt, black pepper, paprika, and oregano.

2. Then, cook the steaks on the preheated grill, turning them over once or twice. Cook for about 10 minutes or until slightly charred.

3. Cut the beef into strips and then place them in a salad bowl. Add in the remaining ingredients, except for the pita; toss to combine well.

4. Top your salad with the toasted pita and serve. Bon appétit!

Nutrition:

Calories: 485 Fat: 39.3g Carbs: 13g Protein: 23.3g

39. Herb and Wine Beef Stew

Preparation Time: 5 minutes

Cooking Time: 55 minutes

Servings: 4

Ingredients

- 2 tbsp. olive oil

- Sea salt

- Freshly ground black pepper, to taste

- 1 tsp. smoked paprika

- 2 pounds beef stew meat, boneless and cut into bite-sized cubes

- One red onion, chopped

- 1 pound Yukon Gold potatoes, peeled and diced

- Two carrots, sliced

- Three cloves garlic, minced

- Two tomatoes, pureed

- 2 cups beef bone broth

- 1/2 cup dry red wine

- Two bay leaves

- Two thyme sprigs

- Two rosemary sprigs

Directions

1. Heat the olive oil in a heavy-bottomed pot over a medium-high flame. Once hot, sear the meat for about 4 minutes until no longer pink; reserve.

2. Season the meat with salt, black pepper, and smoked paprika.

3. Add in the vegetables and continue sautéing for about 5 minutes or until they are crisp-tender.

4. Put the meat back to the pot along with the pureed tomatoes, beef bone broth, red wine, bay leaves, thyme, and rosemary. Bring to a boil and immediately reduce the heat to a simmer.

5. Let it simmer, partially covered, for about 50 minutes or until everything is cooked through.

6. Ladle into individual bowls. Bon appétit!

Nutrition:

Calories: 481 Fat: 16.8g

Carbs: 27.1g

Protein: 55.4g

40.   Classic Italian Stir-Fry

Preparation Time: 5 minutes

Cooking Time: 11 minutes

Servings: 3

Ingredients

- 2 tbsp. olive oil

- 3/4 pound beef brisket, cut into bite-sized strips

- 2 Italian peppers, sliced

- 1 cup cauliflower florets

- One red onion, sliced

- 1 cup brown Italian mushrooms, sliced

- One medium zucchini, julienned

- Two garlic cloves, sliced

- 1/2 tsp. dried basil

- 1 tsp. dried oregano

- 1/2 tsp. crushed red pepper flakes

- Salt and ground black pepper, to taste

- 1/2 cup Greek olives, pitted and sliced

Directions

1. In a prepared large skillet, heat the olive oil until sizzling. Then, stir-fry the beef for about 5 minutes until no longer pink. Place the meat to one side of the skillet.

2. Add in the peppers, cauliflower, and onion and continue to cook for 3 minutes more.

3. Now, stir in the mushrooms, zucchini, garlic, basil, oregano, red pepper flakes, salt, and black pepper; stir-fry for a further 3 minutes or until the vegetables are just tender and fragrant.

4. Top with the olives and serve warm. Bon appétit!

Nutrition:

Calories: 369 Fat: 28.5g Carbs: 10.1g Protein: 19.4g

41.   Beef Salad with Green Beans

Preparation Time: 10 minutes

Cooking Time: 10 minutes

Servings: 4

Ingredients

- 3/4 pound beef tenderloin, fat trimmed, sliced

- Sea salt to taste Ground black pepper, to taste

- 1/2 tsp. red pepper flakes, crushed

- 1 tbsp. olive oil

- 1/2 tsp. dried oregano

- 1/2 tsp. dried rosemary

- 1/2 pound green beans

- One red onion, sliced

- One garlic clove, minced

- 1 Persian cucumber, sliced

- One tomato, sliced

- Two roasted peppers, deseeded and sliced

- One green bell pepper, sliced

- 2 tbsp. fresh parsley, roughly chopped

- 2 tbsp. fresh basil, roughly chopped

- 2 tbsp. fresh mint leaves, roughly chopped

- 1 tbsp. lemon juice

- 4 tbsp. extra-virgin olive oil

- 2 cups butterhead lettuce

- 2 cups baby spinach

Directions

1. Place the green bean in a saucepan and cover it with cold water (2 inches above them). Bring to a boil and turn the heat to a simmer.

2. Let it simmer for about 5 minutes or until they are crisp-tender; drain the green bean; place them in a bowl of the ice water; drain and reserve.

3. Sprinkle the salt, black pepper, and red pepper evenly over the steaks. Heat the olive oil in a cast-iron skillet over a high flame.

4. Once hot, cook the stakes for 3 to 4 minutes per side or until browned. Reduce the heat to medium-low; add in the oregano and rosemary and continue to sauté an additional 30 seconds or until fragrant.

5. Cut the steaks into strips and transfer them to a salad bowl. Add in the remaining ingredients and toss to coat.

6. Top with the green beans. Bon appétit!

Nutrition:

Calories: 434

Fat: 35.3g

Carbs: 10.5g

Protein: 18.4g

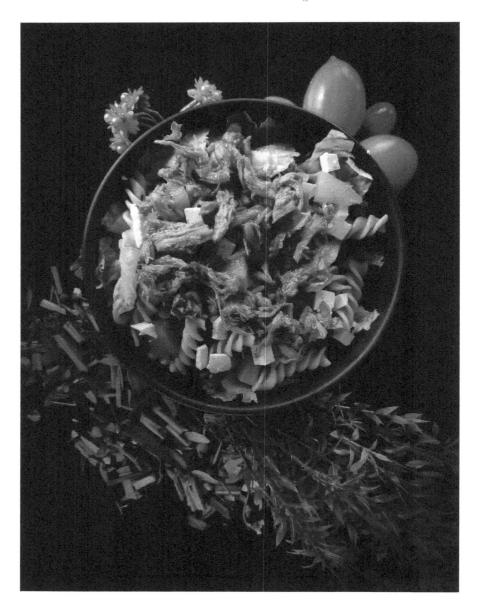

CHAPTER 9:

Vegetable

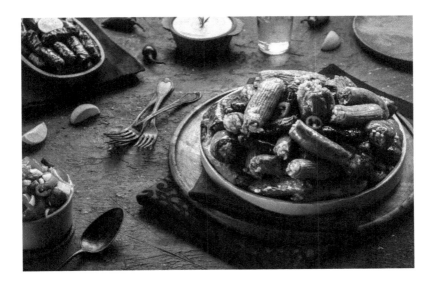

42.　Rosemary-Roasted Red Potatoes

Preparation Time: 5 minutes

Cooking Time: 20 minutes

Servings: 6

Ingredients:

- 1 pound red potatoes, quartered

- ¼ cup olive oil

- ½ tsp. kosher salt

- ¼ tsp. black pepper

- One garlic clove, minced

- Four rosemary sprigs

Directions:

1. Preheat the air fryer to 360°F.

2. In a large bowl, toss the potatoes with olive oil, salt, pepper, and garlic until well coated.

3. Pour the potatoes into the air fryer basket and top with the sprigs of rosemary.

4. Roast for 10 minutes, then stir or toss the potatoes and roast for 10 minutes more.

5. Remove the rosemary sprigs and serve the potatoes. Season with additional salt and pepper, if needed.

Nutrition:

Calories: 133

Fat: 9g

Protein: 1g

Carbohydrates: 12g

43. Roasted Radishes with Sea Salt

Preparation: 5 minutes Cooking: 18 minutes   Servings: 4

Ingredients:

- 1 pound radishes, ends trimmed if needed

- 2 tbsp. olive oil

- ½ tsp. sea salt

Directions:

1. Preheat the air fryer to 360°F.

2. In a large bowl, combine the radishes with olive oil and sea salt.

3. Pour the radishes into the air fryer and cook for 10 minutes. Stir or turn the radishes over and cook for 8 minutes more, then serve.

Nutrition:

Calories: 78 Fat: 9g

Protein: 1g Carbohydrates: 4g Fiber: 2g

44.   Garlic Zucchini and Red Peppers

Preparation: 5 minutes Cooking: 15 minutes   Servings: 6

Ingredients:

- Two medium zucchini, cubed

- One red bell pepper, diced

- Two garlic cloves, sliced

- 2 tbsp. olive oil ½ tsp. salt

Directions:

1. Preheat the air fryer to 380°F.

2. In a large bowl, mix the zucchini, bell pepper, and garlic with olive oil and salt.

3. Pour the mixture into the air fryer basket, and roast for 7 minutes. Shake or stir, then burn for 7 to 8 minutes more.

Nutrition:

Calories: 60 Fat: 5g Protein: 1g Carbohydrates: 4g

Fiber: 1g

45.   Parmesan and Herb Sweet Potatoes

Preparation Time: 10 minutes

Cooking Time: 18 minutes

Servings: 4

Ingredients:

- Two large sweet potatoes, peeled and cubed

- ¼ cup olive oil

- 1 tsp. dried rosemary

- ½ tsp. salt

- 2 tbsp. shredded Parmesan

Directions:

1. Preheat the air fryer to 360°F.

2. In a large bowl, toss the sweet potatoes with olive oil, rosemary, and salt.

3. Pour the potatoes into the air fryer basket and roast for 10 minutes, then stir the potatoes and sprinkle the

Parmesan over the top. Continue roasting for 8 minutes more.

4. Serve hot and enjoy.

Nutrition:

Calories: 186

 Fat: 14g

Protein: 2g

Carbohydrates: 13g

Fiber: 2g

46. Roasted Brussels sprouts with Orange and Garlic

Preparation Time: 5 minutes

Cooking Time: 10 minutes

Servings: 4

Ingredients:

- 1 pound Brussels sprouts, quartered

- Two garlic cloves, minced

- 2 tbsp. olive oil

- ½ tsp. salt

- One orange, cut into rings

Directions:

1. Preheat the air fryer to 360°F.

2. In a large bowl, toss the quartered Brussels sprouts with garlic, olive oil, and salt until well coated.

3. Pour the Brussels sprouts into the air fryer, lay the orange slices on top of them, and roast for 10 minutes.

4. Remove from the air fryer and set the orange slices aside. Toss the Brussels sprouts before serving.

Nutrition:

Calories: 111

Fat: 7g

Protein: 4g

Carbohydrates: 11g

Fiber: 4g

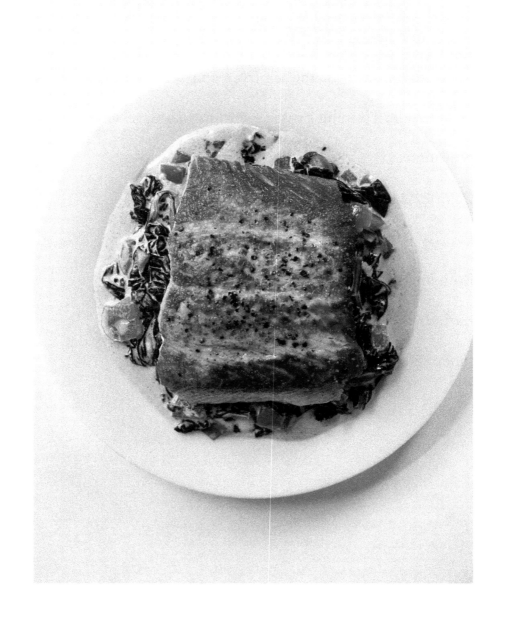

CHAPTER 10:

Desserts

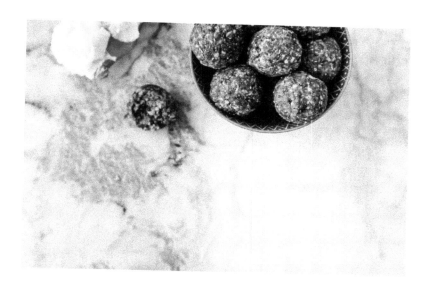

47. Baked Apples with Walnuts and Spices

Preparation Time: 10 minutes

Cooking Time: 45 minutes

Servings: 4

Ingredients:

- Four apples

- ¼ cup chopped walnuts

- 2 tbsp. honey

- 1 tsp. ground cinnamon

- ¼ tsp. ground nutmeg

- ¼ tsp. ground ginger

- Pinch sea salt

Directions:

1. Preheat the oven to 375°F.

2. Cut the tops off the apples and then use a metal spoon or a paring knife to remove the cores, leaving

the bottoms of the apples intact. Place the apples cut-side up in a 9-by-9-inch baking pan.

3. Stir together the walnuts, honey, cinnamon, nutmeg, ginger, and sea salt. Put the mixture into the centers of the apples. Bake the apples for about 45 minutes until browned, soft, and fragrant. Serve warm.

Nutrition:

Calories: 199

Carbohydrates: 41g

Protein: 5g

Fat: 5g

48.   Vanilla Pudding with Strawberries

Preparation Time: 10 minutes

Cooking Time: 10 minutes + chilling time

Servings: 4

Ingredients:

- 2¼ cups skim milk, divided

- One egg, beaten

- ½ cup sugar

- 1 tsp. vanilla extract

- Pinch sea salt

- 3 tbsp. cornstarch

- 2 cups sliced strawberries

Directions:

1. In a small bowl, whisk 2 cups of milk with the egg, sugar, vanilla, and sea salt. Transfer the mixture to a

medium pot, place it over medium heat, and slowly bring to a boil, whisking constantly.

2. Whisk the cornstarch with ¼ cup of milk. In a thin stream, whisk this slurry into the boiling mixture in the pot. Cook until it thickens, stirring constantly. Boil for 1 minute more, stirring constantly.

3. Spoon the pudding into four dishes and refrigerate to chill. Serve topped with the sliced strawberries.

Nutrition:

Calories: 209

Carbohydrates: 43g

Protein: 6g

Fat: 1g

49. Mixed Berry Frozen Yogurt Bar

Preparation Time: 10 minutes

Cooking Time: 0 minutes

Servings: 8

Ingredients:

- 8 cups low-fat vanilla frozen yogurt (or flavor of choice)

- 1 cup sliced fresh strawberries

- 1 cup fresh blueberries

- 1 cup fresh blackberries

- 1 cup fresh raspberries

- ½ cup chopped walnuts

Directions:

1. Apportion the yogurt among eight dessert bowls.

2. Serve the toppings family-style, and let your guests choose their toppings and spoon them over the yogurt.

Nutrition:

Calories: 81 Carbohydrates: 9g Protein: 3g

Fat: 5g

50. Cherry Brownies with Walnuts

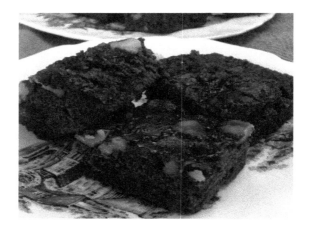

Preparation Time: 10 minutes

Cooking Time: 25-30 minutes

Servings: 9

Ingredients:

- Nine fresh cherries that are stemmed and pitted or nine frozen cherries

- ½ cup sugar or sweetener substitute

- ¼ cup extra virgin olive oil

- 1 tsp. vanilla extract

- ¼ tsp. sea salt

- ½ cup whole-wheat pastry flour

- ¼ tsp. baking powder

- 1/3 cup walnuts, chopped

- Two eggs

- ½ cup plain Greek yogurt

- 1/3 cup cocoa powder, unsweetened

Directions:

1. Make sure one of the metal racks in your oven is set in the middle.

2. Turn the temperature on your oven to 375 degrees Fahrenheit.

3. Using cooking spray, grease a 9-inch square pan.

4. Take a large bowl and add the oil and sugar or sweetener substitute. Whisk the ingredients well.

5. Add the eggs and use a mixer to beat the ingredients together.

6. Pour in the yogurt and continue to beat the mixture until it is smooth.

7. Take a medium bowl and combine the cocoa powder, flour, sea salt, and baking powder by whisking them together.

8. Combine the powdered ingredients into the wet ingredients and use your electronic mixer to thoroughly incorporate the ingredients together.

9. Add in the walnuts and stir.

10. Pour the mixture into the pan.

11. Sprinkle the cherries on top and push them into the batter. You can use any design, but it is best to make three rows and three columns with the cherries. This ensures that each piece of the brownie will have one cherry.

12. Put the batter into the oven and turn your timer to 20 minutes.

13. Check that the brownies are done using the toothpick test before removing them from the oven. Push the toothpick into the middle of the brownies and once it comes out clean, remove the brownies.

14. Let the brownies cool for 5 to 10 minutes before cutting and serving.

Nutrition:

Calories: 225 Fats: 10 grams

Carbohydrates: 30 grams

Protein: 5 grams.

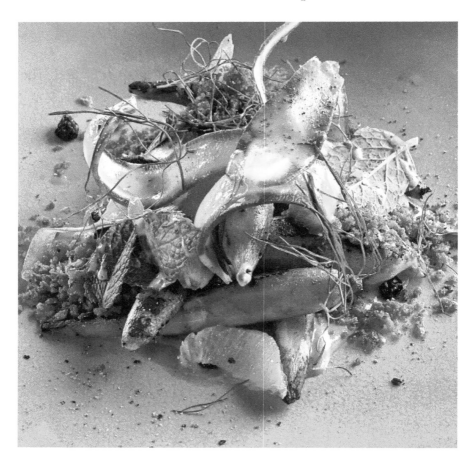

30 Day Meal Plan

Days	Breakfast	Lunch	Dinner	Snacks
1	Banana Nut Oatmeal	Mediterranean Spaghetti	Chicken Wrap	Walnuts Yogurt Dip
2	Greek Yogurt Pancakes	Chicken With Peas	Rosemary-Roasted Red Potatoes	Creamy Pepper Spread
3	Omelet Provencale	Caprese Pasta Salad	Lemon Herb Potatoes	Perfect Queso
4	Chili Cheese Omelet	Sautéed Cabbage With Parsley	Almond Chicken Bites	Fluffy Bites
5	Strawberry Marmalade	Mushroom And Garlic Spaghetti	Baked Salmon With Tarragon Mustard Sauce	Coconut Fudge
6	Avocado Breakfast Sandwiches	Greek Green Beans	Baked Lemon Salmon	Tasty Black Bean Dip
7	Greek Yogurt Parfait	One-Pan Tuscan Chicken	Baby Kale And Cabbage Salad	Cucumber Tomato Okra Salsa
8	Yogurt Cheese	Tomato Pasta Fagioli	Chicken And Black Beans	Cheesy Corn Dip
9	Arugula Frittata	Delicious Pepper Zucchini	Halibut And Quinoa Mix	Chili Mango And Watermelon Salsa
10	Sweet Oatmeal	Celery Carrot	Lemon and	Yogurt Dip

		Brown Lentils	Dates Barramundi	
11	Avocado Toast	Catfish Fillets And Rice	Halibut And Quinoa Mix	Slow-Cooked Cheesy Artichoke Dip
12	Baked Eggs With Parsley	Pasta With Creamy Sauce	Butter Chicken Thighs	cucumber sandwich bites
13	Yogurt With Dates	Feta Macaroni	Parmesan Chicken	Rosemary Hummus
14	Artichoke Omelet	Pecan Salmon Fillets	Turkey And Cranberry Sauce	Sausage Queso Dip
15	Banana Oats	Salmon and Broccoli	Parmesan-Thyme Butternut Squash	Yogurt Dip
16	Sun-Dried Tomatoes Oatmeal	Turkey Burgers With Mango Salsa	Cod and Mushrooms Mix	Nutmeg Nougat
17	Berry Oats	Crispy Garlic Sliced Eggplant	Chicken and Olives Salsa	Sweet Almond Bites
18	Greek Yogurt Parfait	Basil Buckwheat Pasta	Chili Chicken Mix	Walnuts Yogurt Dip
19	Banana Quinoa	Parmesan and Herb Sweet Potatoes	Salmon And Peach Pan	Flavorful Italian Peppers
20	Greek Yogurt W/Berries & Seeds	Crispy Lemon Artichoke Hearts	Garlic Zucchini And Red Peppers	Cheese Stuff Artichokes
21	Mediterranean Diet Breakfast Tostadas	Citrus Green Beans With Red Onions	Feta Green Beans	Walnuts Yogurt Dip
22	Greek Yogurt	Sesame	Healthy	Flavorful

	W/Berries & Seeds	Shrimp Mix	Vegetable Medley	Roasted Baby Potatoes
23	Yogurt Cheese	Baked Shrimp Mix	Flavors Basil Lemon Ratatouille	Cucumber Rolls
24	Chickpea Soup With Shrimp	Shrimp And Lemon Sauce	Garlic Basil Zucchini	Olives And Cheese Stuffed Tomatoes
25	Creamy Loaded Mashed Potatoes	Cauliflower Rice	Baked Halibut Steaks With Vegetables	Mixed Berry Frozen Yogurt Bar
26	Mediterranean Egg Scramble	Bacon Linguine Pasta	Turkey, Artichokes and Asparagus	Veggie Fritters
27	Avocado Green Apple Breakfast Smoothie	Tomato Dill Cauliflower	Double Cheesy Bacon Chicken	Wrapped Plums
28	Breakfast Toast	Parsnips With Eggplant	Crispy Italian Chicken	Bulgur Lamb Meatballs
29	Savory Egg Galettes	Halibut Roulade	Olive Oil Poached Cod	Almond Shortbread Cookies
30	Spinach Frittata	Chicken And Butter Sauce	Pistachio-Crusted Halibut	Crunchy Sesame Cookies

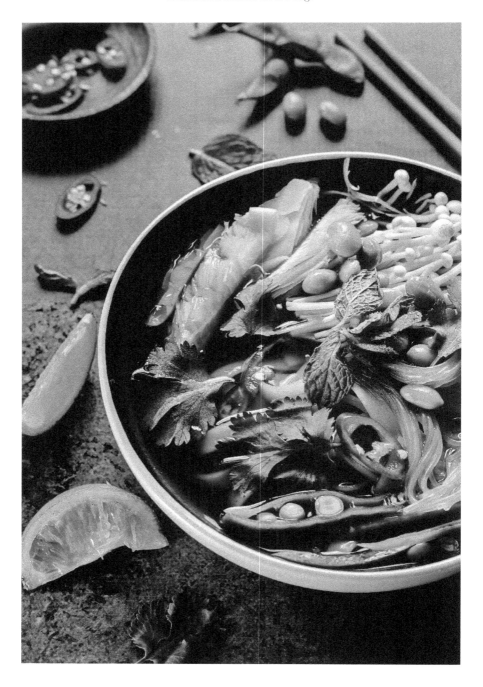

Conclusion:

Thank you for reading the Mediterranean Diet cookbook. The recipes and ideas in this book help you and your family. Mediterranean diet is known to be good for your heart. The key to a healthy diet is variety. Eat a variety of foods from various food groups each day. Make half your grain products whole-grain each day. Make at least three servings of vegetables and fruits and at least two servings of milk each day. The recipes in this book all have healthy fats that help lower bad cholesterol while preventing heart attacks. Some of the recipes may be higher in calories than other diet dishes, but these healthy oils are very beneficial to your cholesterol normalization. Greek yogurt provides mucus relief to your body. Healthy fats such as avocados are very helpful. Avocados contain healthier fats than any other vegetable source. The recipes in this book use only one-third of an avocado to provide the right amount of healthy fats. The Mediterranean diet also regulates your insulin levels to normalize your blood sugar consumption. This is the key to a healthy diet. Once you have balanced your blood sugar, your body will be in a stable state for the rest of your life.

Consuming the Mediterranean diet minimalizes the use of processed foods. It has been related to a reduced level of risk in developing numerous chronic diseases, decreased risk of obesity, diabetes, coronary artery disease, and cognitive impairment, which are all included in these benefits. The Mediterranean diet is generally associated with highly-spiced dishes that involve little or no cooking. They are generally made up of fresh ingredients out of doors, including substantial use of nuts, fruits, vegetables, and fish. Consuming alkaline foods such as vegetables and herbs for seasoning is another major aspect of the diet that brings about an alkalinity to the body. Most people trying the Mediterranean diet have gained positive results in cutting their weight. These positive results include a reduction in the excess fat, along with the loss of abdominal skin, and a reduction in blood pressure. When you go for a Mediterranean diet, the body moves towards a sustainable model that burns calories slowly. When you ingest foods and drinks that contain more of the natural oils, it significantly reduces the absorption of the carbohydrates that are found in foods. You will also consume foods with less fat, which is better for the absorption of the nutrients that your body needs. People, who don't have carbohydrate intolerance problems, can successfully use this diet. One great aspect of this diet is that it is not all about the meat, but rather it also involves fruit, fish, and vegetables. Meat only accounts for about a third of the Mediterranean food group. Some of the benefits that this diet will offer you are a reduction in abdominal fat, heartbeat irregularities, and decreased blood sugar. Moving on, you can easily see how a Mediterranean diet would be invaluable for many people's well-being. The comprehensive lifestyle change that would most likely benefit you is that it will instantly improve your overall health and well-being. Â Apart from the healing effects that you will experience, the life-extension aspect is also a plus. So, it's becoming more and more appealing to many, due to the benefits that it offers. It is one of the most beneficial diets to avoid cardiovascular diseases. It is rich in nuts and rich anti-inflammatory benefits that help people who eat Mediterranean type foods.

CPSIA information can be obtained
at www.ICGtesting.com
Printed in the USA
BVHW052043210721
612428BV00002B/58